THE ART OF TAKING ACTION

THE ART OF TAKING ACTION

Empower Your Life

COACH JOHN BEZERRA

John Bezerra

Table of Contents

Table of Contents

Introduction

Introduction: The Power of Taking Action and Overcoming Inaction

In the grand theater of life, there exists a pivotal force, often underestimated, yet profoundly transformative—the power of action. It is a force that propels us forward, transforms dreams into reality, and bridges the vast chasm between where we are and where we aspire to be. But within the shadow of this force, there lurks a formidable adversary—inaction, the silent saboteur of dreams.

Each of us harbors aspirations, ambitions, and desires. We envision better versions of ourselves, dream of accomplishments yet to be unlocked, and yearn for lives rich in purpose and fulfillment. These dreams are the seeds of our potential, the sparks of our creativity, and the essence of our happiness. Yet, too often, they remain dormant, smothered beneath layers of doubt, fear, and procrastination.

In this exploration of the power of taking action and the art of overcoming inaction, we embark on a journey of self-discovery and transformation. We delve deep into the intricate workings of our minds and hearts, seeking to unravel the mysteries that hold us back and uncover the hidden springs of motivation that can propel us forward.

This journey is not a mere intellectual exercise but a call to action—a call to embrace the full potential of our lives. It's an invitation to step onto the stage, to take center stage in our own stories, and to become the authors of our destinies. It's a reminder that inaction is not the path to fulfillment, but rather, it's the bold steps we take, the decisions we make, and the persistence we exhibit that lead us toward the life we desire.

Throughout these pages, we will explore the psychology behind inaction, learn the art of setting clear and compelling goals, and master the strategies to conquer fear, doubt, and procrastination. We will discover the exhilaration of that initial step and the steady rhythm of consistent action. We will also explore the role of accountability, the importance of celebrating progress, and the transformative potential of embracing change.

As we venture forth on this quest, let us remember that it is not the absence of challenges that defines us, but rather, it is our ability to rise above them. The power of taking action lies within each of us, waiting to be harnessed and directed toward our deepest desires. Together, we will unlock that power, illuminate the path forward, and embark on a journey toward a life filled with purpose, passion, and achievement.

Chapter 1: The Psychology of Procrastination and Identifying Your Personal Barriers

Procrastination, that seemingly innocuous thief of time, has plagued humanity since time immemorial. We've all been there—faced with tasks that need attention, deadlines looming, yet we find ourselves irresistibly drawn to distractions, delaying the inevitable. Understanding the psychology behind procrastination and recognizing the unique barriers that hinder our progress is the first step in overcoming this pervasive challenge.

The Procrastination Paradox

Procrastination is paradoxical in nature. It provides temporary relief from stress and anxiety, yet it compounds our long-term challenges. To conquer it, we must first understand why we procrastinate:

-

**Instant Gratification**: Our brains are wired to seek immediate rewards. Procrastination often offers the promise of instant gratification, such as scrolling through social media or watching TV, which feels more appealing than tackling a daunting task.

Fear of Failure: Procrastination can be a defense mechanism against fear of failure. By delaying a task, we avoid the possibility of falling short and facing disappointment.

Lack of Motivation: When a task lacks intrinsic motivation or feels overwhelming, we tend to postpone it. The absence of clear goals or enthusiasm can lead to chronic procrastination.

Perfectionism: The desire for perfection can paralyze us. Procrastinators often set unrealistically high standards, fearing they won't meet them and thus never start.

Time Discounting: We often undervalue future rewards and overvalue immediate comfort. This leads to choices that favor short-term pleasure over long-term gains.

Identifying Your Personal Procrastination Barriers

Procrastination is a deeply personal challenge, and its roots can vary from person to person. To combat it effectively, we must identify our unique barriers:

- *Self-Reflection*: Take time to reflect on your procrastination patterns. Are there specific types of tasks or situations where you tend to procrastinate more?

- *Triggers*: What external or internal triggers lead you to procrastinate? Stress, boredom, or lack of interest can all be triggers.

- *Excuses*: What excuses do you use to justify procrastination? Recognizing these rationalizations is crucial for change.

- *Emotions*: Pay attention to the emotions associated with procrastination. Anxiety, guilt, or a sense of being overwhelmed are common emotional triggers.

- *Time Management*: Assess your time management skills. Are you allocating time effectively to your tasks, or is poor time management contributing to procrastination?

In this chapter, we'll explore practical strategies to address these barriers and develop a personalized action plan. By unraveling the psychology of procrastination and gaining insight into our individual hurdles, we pave the way for effective solutions and a more productive, fulfilled life. Remember, conquering procrastination is not just about managing time; it's about mastering your mind.

Procrastination Traits Worksheet

Procrastination is a common challenge, and understanding your specific procrastination traits is the first step toward overcoming them. In this worksheet, we will identify and explore five key procrastination traits mentioned in Chapter 1: The Psychology of Procrastination.

Trait *1*: *Instant Gratification*

Think about tasks you often delay. What activities or distractions do you turn to when avoiding these tasks? List them below.
- Distraction 1:
- Distraction 2:
- Distraction 3:

Trait 2: *Fear of Failure*

Reflect on a recent task you procrastinated on. Did fear of failure play a role in your procrastination? If so, describe how.
- Task:
- Fear of Failure Impact:

Trait 3: *Lack of Motivation*

Consider a task you've been putting off. Is it because you lack motivation or enthusiasm for it? Describe the task and your feelings toward it.
- Task:
- Lack of Motivation:

<u>**Trait 4**: *Perfectionism*</u>

Think about a project where you aimed for perfection. Did this desire for perfection lead to procrastination? Describe the project and your perfectionist tendencies.

- Project:
- Perfectionism Impact:

-

<u>**Trait 5**: *Time Discounting*</u>

Recall a situation where you chose short-term comfort over long-term benefits. What task or responsibility did you delay, and what immediate comfort did you opt for instead?

- Task Delayed:
- Immediate Comfort Chosen:

-

<u>****Self-Reflection:****</u>

Now that you've identified these procrastination traits in your behavior, take a moment to reflect:

- Which trait(s) seem to be the most significant contributors to your procrastination?
- Are there any common patterns or recurring themes in your procrastination habits?
- How do these traits impact your productivity, goals, and overall well-being?

Recognizing these procrastination traits is an important step toward overcoming procrastination. In the following chapters of this guide, we will delve deeper into strategies and techniques to address each of these traits and empower you to take action in your life.

Remember, overcoming procrastination is a journey, and self-awareness is your compass. By understanding your procrastination tendencies, you are already on the path to change and personal growth.

Chapter 2: The Importance of Goal Setting and 5 SMART Goals

Goals are the compass that guides us through the labyrinth of life. They give us direction, purpose, and the motivation to take action. In this chapter, we'll explore the profound significance of goal setting and introduce you to the concept of SMART goals—specific, measurable, achievable, relevant, and time-bound.

The Power of Goals

Goals are like beacons on the horizon, illuminating the path we wish to tread. Here's why they matter:

-

Clarity of Purpose: Goals provide clarity about what you want to achieve. They transform vague desires into concrete objectives.

-

Motivation and Focus: Goals ignite motivation. They give you a reason to wake up each morning with determination and provide a focal point for your efforts.

-

<u>Measuring Progress</u>: Goals enable you to track your progress. They help you assess how far you've come and what remains to be done.

<u>Overcoming Procrastination</u>: Setting deadlines and milestones associated with goals can combat procrastination, as it provides a sense of urgency.

Now, let's delve into SMART goals—an approach that ensures your goals are well-defined and actionable.

The SMART Goal Framework

S - Specific: Your goal should be crystal clear and specific. Avoid vague aspirations. Ask yourself: What exactly do I want to accomplish?

M - Measurable: Goals should be quantifiable. How will you measure your progress and know when you've achieved your goal? Define specific metrics.

A - Achievable: Goals should be realistic and attainable. While aiming high is admirable, ensure your goals are within your reach with effort and commitment.

R - Relevant: The goal should be aligned with your values, priorities, and long-term objectives. Does it make sense in the context of your life?

T - Time-Bound: Set a deadline. Without a timeframe, a goal is just a wish. When do you intend to achieve this goal?

Now, let's put theory into practice. Create five SMART goals that reflect different aspects of your life. These goals should be specific, measurable, achievable, relevant, and time-bound.

1. *Professional Goal:*
   - S - What is the specific career achievement you're targeting?
   - M - How will you measure your progress?
   - A - Is it realistically attainable?
   - R - Does it align with your career aspirations?
   - T - Set a deadline for this goal.
2. *Personal Development Goal*:
   - S - What skill or personal growth area do you want to focus on?
   - M - How will you measure your improvement?
   - A - Can you realistically commit to this?
   - R - Does it align with your personal values?
   - T - Set a timeframe for achieving this goal.
3. *Health and Wellness Goal*:
   - S - What specific aspect of your health are you targeting?
   - M - How will you measure your progress?
   - A - Is it achievable given your current circumstances?
   - R - Does it align with your overall well-being?
   - T - Set a deadline for this health goal.
4. *Financial Goal:*
   - S - What financial milestone are you aiming for?
   - M - How will you measure your financial progress?
   - A - Is it within your financial means?
   - R - Does it align with your long-term financial plans?
   - T - Specify the timeframe for achieving this financial goal.

5.Relationship Goal:
- S - What specific improvement or change do you want in a relationship?
- M - How will you measure progress in the relationship?
- A - Is this goal realistic within the context of the relationship?
- R - Does it align with your values and the health of the relationship?
- T - Set a deadline for achieving this relationship goal.

By crafting these five SMART goals, you're taking a significant step toward turning your aspirations into tangible, achievable outcomes. Goals bring your vision to life, and the SMART framework ensures they are well-defined and actionable. In the upcoming chapters, we'll explore strategies for planning and executing these goals effectively.

Chapter 3: Creating an Action Plan, Prioritization, and Time Management

Goals are the stars that guide our journey, but without a roadmap, they remain distant dreams. In this chapter, we will dive into the crucial steps of creating a concrete action plan, mastering the art of prioritization, and honing your time management skills to transform your goals into reality.

Creating Your Action Plan

An action plan is the bridge that connects your goals to the actions required to achieve them. Here's how to create one:

- **Break It Down**: Divide your goal into smaller, manageable tasks. This simplifies the journey, making it less daunting.

- **Set Deadlines**: Assign deadlines to each task. Deadlines create a sense of urgency and accountability.

__Prioritize__: Decide which tasks are most critical to your goal's success and order them accordingly.

__Allocate Resources__: Determine what resources you need, whether it's time, money, or skills.

__Measure Progress__: Establish checkpoints to measure your progress along the way.

Mastering Prioritization

Prioritization is the art of distinguishing between what's important and what's urgent. To prioritize effectively:

-

**Eisenhower Matrix**:

Use this tool to categorize tasks into four quadrants:
- Important and Urgent: Do these tasks immediately.
- Important but Not Urgent: Plan and schedule these tasks.
- Urgent but Not Important: Delegate these tasks if possible.
- Not Urgent and Not Important: Consider eliminating or postponing these tasks.

-

**ABC Method**:

Label tasks as A (most important), B (important), or C (less important). Focus on A tasks first.

-

**Value vs. Effort**:

Assess the value and effort required for each task. Prioritize those with high value and reasonable effort.

Effective Time Management

Time is your most valuable resource. To manage it effectively:

- ***Set Clear Boundaries***: Establish specific work hours and personal time to maintain a healthy work-life balance.

- ***Use Time Blocks***: Allocate dedicated time blocks for specific tasks or categories of work.

- ***Minimize Distractions***: Identify common distractions and develop strategies to minimize them.

- ***Utilize Technology***: Use productivity apps and tools to track time and manage tasks.

- ***Regular Breaks***: Take short, scheduled breaks to recharge and maintain focus.

Your Action Plan:

Now, let's put these principles into practice. Create an action plan for one of the SMART goals you defined in Chapter 2. Follow these steps:

- *Goal*: Write down the SMART goal you want to work on.

- *Task Breakdown*: List the specific tasks required to achieve this goal.

- *Deadlines*: Assign deadlines to each task.

- *Prioritization*: Determine the priority of each task using the techniques mentioned earlier.

- *Resources*: Identify any resources or support you need for each task.

- *Progress Checkpoints*: Set checkpoints or milestones to measure your progress.

- *Time Blocks*: Allocate specific time blocks in your schedule for working on these tasks.

By creating this action plan, you're not just setting intentions—you're taking concrete steps toward achieving your goals. In the following chapters, we'll delve deeper into strategies for overcoming common obstacles, staying motivated, and adapting your plan as needed. Remember, action plans coupled with effective prioritization and time management can turn even the loftiest goals into attainable targets.

Chapter 4: Overcoming Fear and Doubt, Tackling Fear of Failure, and Building Self-Confidence

Fear and doubt are formidable adversaries on the path to success. In this chapter, we'll explore strategies to conquer these inner obstacles, particularly the fear of failure, and bolster your self-confidence as you pursue your goals with resilience and determination.

Understanding Fear and Doubt

Fear and doubt are natural emotions, but when left unaddressed, they can paralyze us. Here's how to understand and manage them:

-

Identify Triggers: Recognize situations or thoughts that trigger fear and doubt. Understanding your triggers is the first step to managing them effectively.

-

Analyze Your Fears: Ask yourself what you're truly afraid of. Often, our fears are based on irrational beliefs. Challenge these beliefs with logic and evidence.

-

Acceptance: Understand that everyone experiences fear and doubt at times. It's a part of being human. Accepting these feelings can reduce their power over you.

Tackling Fear of Failure

The fear of failure is one of the most common barriers to taking action. Here's how to confront it:

-

Reframe Failure: Shift your perspective on failure. Instead of seeing it as a negative outcome, view it as a valuable learning experience.

-

Set Realistic Expectations: Understand that not every endeavor will lead to success, and that's okay. Set realistic expectations for yourself.

-

Break Tasks Down: Divide your goals into smaller tasks. This makes failure in one aspect less daunting and allows for incremental progress.

-

Visualize Success: Use visualization techniques to picture yourself succeeding. This can boost your confidence and reduce fear.

Building Self-Confidence

Self-confidence is the antidote to self-doubt. Here's how to cultivate it:

-

Acknowledge Your Achievements: Reflect on past successes, no matter how small. Recognize your abilities and strengths.

-

Positive Self-Talk: Replace self-criticism with positive affirmations. Challenge negative thoughts and replace them with constructive ones.

-

Expand Your Comfort Zone: Step out of your comfort zone regularly. Each small success will boost your confidence.

-

Set Achievable Goals: Start with goals you know you can accomplish. As you achieve them, your confidence will grow.

Your Fear and Confidence Action Plan:

Now, let's put these principles into action. Choose one goal from your list of SMART goals in Chapter 2. This should be a goal that you've hesitated to pursue due to fear or self-doubt.

- *Goal*: Write down the SMART goal you've chosen.

- *Identify Fear and Doubt*: Describe the specific fears and doubts that have held you back from pursuing this goal.

- *Reframe Fear of Failure*: Apply the techniques mentioned earlier to reframe your fear of failure for this goal.

- *Boost Self-Confidence*: List three actions you can take to boost your self-confidence in relation to this goal.

- *Create a Fear-Action Plan*: Outline specific steps you will take to confront and overcome your fear or doubts related to this goal.

- *Visualize Success*: Spend a few minutes visualizing yourself achieving this goal. Imagine the positive emotions and sense of accomplishment.

By completing this action plan, you'll equip yourself with the tools to face your fears, overcome self-doubt, and build the self-confidence necessary to pursue your goals with renewed vigor. In the following chapters, we'll continue to explore strategies for staying resilient and maintaining your confidence as you take action in your life.

Chapter 5: Taking the First Step - The Momentum of Initial Action and Cultivating a Bias for Action

The first step is often the most challenging, yet it holds the key to unlocking a cascade of momentum. In this chapter, we'll explore the significance of taking that initial leap, harnessing the power of momentum, and nurturing a natural inclination for action.

The Paralysis of Inaction

Procrastination thrives in the realm of inaction. It feeds on hesitation and doubt, keeping us trapped in a cycle of inertia. To break free, we must understand the psychology of that first step:

-

Analysis Paralysis: Overthinking and excessive planning can paralyze us. The initial step is about doing, not just thinking.

-

**The Weight of Perfection**: Aiming for perfection from the outset can be paralyzing. Accept that initial efforts may not be flawless.

-

**The Fear of the Unknown**: Fear often arises from the uncertainty of taking that first step. We tend to imagine worst-case scenarios that rarely come to pass.

The Power of the Initial Action
Taking that first step is like igniting a rocket. Here's why it's so important:

-

**Builds Momentum**: Initial action sets things in motion. Each subsequent step becomes easier as you gain momentum.

-

**Boosts Confidence**: Success in that first step bolsters your confidence. It reinforces the belief that you can achieve your goal.

-

**Creates a Psychological Shift**: It shifts your mindset from contemplation to action. You become an active participant in your journey.

Cultivating a Bias for Action

A bias for action is an innate preference for taking initiative. Here's how to cultivate it:

- ***Set Smaller Goals***: Start with smaller, manageable goals. They require less initial effort and can serve as stepping stones to larger objectives.

- ***Use the 2-Minute Rule**** If a task can be completed in under two minutes, do it immediately. It removes procrastination's grip on minor tasks.

- ***Establish Routines***: Create daily routines that include actions related to your goals. Repetition reinforces the habit of taking action.

- ***Accountability Partners***: Share your goals and progress with a trusted friend or mentor who can hold you accountable for taking action.

Your First Step Action Plan:

Choose one of your SMART goals from Chapter 2. It's time to take that crucial first step. Follow these steps:

- _Goal_: Write down the SMART goal you've selected.

- _**Identify the First Step**_: Determine the very first action you need to take to kickstart progress toward this goal.

- _**Overcome Inertia**_: List any obstacles or doubts that have held you back from taking this initial action.

- _**Set a Date**_: Assign a specific date and time to take this first step.

- _**Visualize Success**_: Spend a few minutes visualizing yourself successfully completing this first step and the positive impact it will have on your journey.

By completing this action plan, you'll break through the inertia that has held you back and begin to experience the exhilarating sensation of progress. Remember, taking the first step is often the most challenging, but it's also the most rewarding. In the upcoming chapters, we'll explore strategies for staying on course and maintaining your momentum.

Chapter 6: Staying Consistent - Building Habits for Long-Term Success and Handling Setbacks and Obstacles

Consistency is the heartbeat of progress, and habits are the foundation upon which it stands. In this chapter, we'll delve into the art of cultivating habits that sustain long-term success and strategies for overcoming setbacks and obstacles along the way.

The Power of Consistency

Consistency turns actions into habits, and habits are the engines of achievement. Here's why consistency matters:

-
Compound Effect: Small, consistent actions accumulate over time, leading to significant results.

-
Reduces Decision Fatigue: Habits remove the need for constant decision-making, preserving mental energy for more critical tasks.

**Fosters Discipline**: Consistency cultivates discipline, enabling you to push through challenges and setbacks.

Building Habits for Success

Building habits is the process of turning intentional actions into automatic behaviors. Here's how to do it effectively:

-

Start Small: Begin with tiny, manageable actions that are easy to integrate into your routine.

-

Consistent Timing: Perform your habit at the same time and in the same context daily.

-

Use Triggers: Associate your habit with an existing routine or trigger, making it easier to remember.

-

Track Progress: Maintain a habit tracker or journal to monitor your consistency.

-

Celebrate Milestones: Acknowledge and reward yourself for achieving milestones in your habit-building journey.

Handling Setbacks and Obstacles

Obstacles and setbacks are inevitable on the path to success. Here's how to navigate them:

-

Resilience: Develop resilience by understanding that setbacks are part of any journey. They provide valuable lessons.

-

Adaptability: Be prepared to adjust your plan when unforeseen circumstances arise.

-

Positive Self-Talk: Use setbacks as opportunities to practice positive self-talk and maintain your confidence.

-

Learn and Pivot: Extract lessons from setbacks and use them to pivot and refine your approach.

<u>Your Consistency and Setback Action Plan:</u>

Choose one of your SMART goals from Chapter 2 and the first step you took in Chapter 5. Now, it's time to turn that first step into a consistent habit and prepare for potential setbacks. Follow these steps:

- **_<u>Goal:</u>_** <u>Write down the SMART goal you've selected.</u>

- **_<u>First Step Habit:</u>_** <u>Identify the initial action you took in Chapter 5 and transform it into a daily or weekly habit.</u>

- **_<u>Habit Building Plan:</u>_** <u>Outline how you will integrate this habit into your daily routine, including the specific time and triggers.</u>

- **_<u>Anticipate Setbacks:</u>_** <u>List potential obstacles or setbacks you might encounter while building this habit.</u>

- **_<u>Contingency Plan:</u>_** <u>Develop strategies to address these setbacks when they occur. How will you adapt and stay on track?</u>

- **_<u>Celebrate Progress:</u>_** <u>Define milestones to celebrate as you build this habit. What rewards or acknowledgments will motivate you?</u>

By completing this action plan, you're creating a framework for building consistent habits that will lead to lasting success. Remember, setbacks are not roadblocks but stepping stones to growth. In the next chapters, we'll explore the role of accountability and celebration in maintaining your momentum and consistency.

Chapter 7: Accountability and Support - Finding Accountability Partners and Seeking Mentorship and Guidance

On the journey towards your goals, you don't have to go it alone. Accountability partners and mentors can provide invaluable support and guidance. In this chapter, we'll explore the significance of accountability and mentorship and how to find the right individuals to support your journey.

The Power of Accountability
Accountability is a potent force that keeps you on track and motivated. Here's why it matters:

-

Commitment: <u>Knowing that someone is tracking your progress can boost your commitment to your goals.</u>

-

**Feedback:** Accountability partners provide constructive feedback and help you course-correct when needed.

-

**Shared Goals:** Partners can share similar goals, creating a sense of camaraderie and mutual motivation.

Finding Accountability Partners

Accountability partners are individuals who share your commitment to personal growth and success. Here's how to find the right accountability partner:

-

**Define Your Needs:** Identify what you expect from an accountability partner. Is it regular check-ins, shared goal setting, or specific expertise?

-

**Network:** Join local or online communities, workshops, or groups related to your goals and interests. These are great places to find potential partners.

-

**Assess Compatibility:** Look for individuals whose goals align with yours and who have a similar level of commitment.

-

**Communication:** Discuss expectations, frequency of check-ins, and how you will hold each other accountable.

The Role of Mentors

Mentors are experienced individuals who provide guidance and wisdom based on their own journeys. Here's why mentorship is invaluable:

-

**Wisdom Transfer**: Mentors can share valuable insights, shortcuts, and lessons learned from their experiences.

-

**Challenge and Growth**: They push you to think beyond your comfort zone and challenge your assumptions.

Inspiration: Mentors can serve as sources of inspiration and motivation.

Seeking Mentorship and Guidance
Finding the right mentor can be a transformative step in your journey. Here's how to seek mentorship effectively:

Clarify Your Goals: Determine what you hope to gain from mentorship and the specific areas in which you need guidance.

Identify Potential Mentors: Look for individuals who have achieved what you aspire to and who align with your values.

Engage Actively: Approach potential mentors respectfully, express your admiration for their work, and explain why you seek their guidance.

Formalize the Relationship: Once you've established a connection, discuss expectations, frequency of meetings, and goals for the mentorship.

Your Accountability and Mentorship Plan:

Now, it's time to take action and find accountability partners and mentors who will support your journey. Follow these steps:

- _Goal:_ Write down the SMART goal you're currently working on.

- _Accountability Partner:_ Identify someone who can serve as your accountability partner for this goal. Explain why you believe they would be a suitable partner.

- _Mentorship:_ Identify a potential mentor who has expertise in the area related to your goal. Share why you admire their work and how their guidance could benefit you.

- _Engagement Plan:_ Outline how you will approach your potential accountability partner and mentor. What specific steps will you take to establish these relationships?

- _Expectations:_ Define your expectations for both the accountability partnership and mentorship. What support and guidance do you hope to receive?

By completing this action plan, you're taking proactive steps to surround yourself with the support and guidance you need to achieve your goals. Accountability partners and mentors can provide valuable perspectives and motivation throughout your journey. In the following chapters, we'll explore strategies for celebrating progress and adapting to change as you move closer to your goals.

Chapter 8: Celebrating Progress - Recognizing Achievements and Maintaining Motivation

Amidst the pursuit of goals, it's crucial to pause and celebrate the journey. In this chapter, we'll explore the significance of recognizing achievements and how to maintain motivation through the ups and downs of your quest.

The Importance of Celebrating Progress
Celebrating progress isn't just about a momentary burst of joy; it's a vital aspect of long-term success. Here's why it's essential:

-

Positive Reinforcement: Celebrating achievements reinforces positive behavior and motivates you to continue striving for your goals.

-

Boosts Confidence: Recognizing your progress bolsters self-confidence, helping you face future challenges with resilience.

-

**Sustains Momentum:** Celebrations inject excitement and energy into your journey, keeping you engaged and enthusiastic.

Effective Ways to Celebrate Progress

Celebrations don't have to be grand or elaborate. They should align with your preferences and your achievements. Here are some ways to celebrate progress effectively:

-

**Set Milestones:** Establish clear milestones for your goals and celebrate when you reach them.

-

**Personal Rewards**: Treat yourself to something you enjoy, whether it's a favorite meal, a movie night, or a small gift.

-

**Share Achievements**: Share your successes with friends, family, or your accountability partner. Let them join in your celebration.

-

**Reflect and Appreciate:** Take time to reflect on the journey and appreciate the effort and dedication you've put in.

Maintaining Motivation

Motivation can wane as you progress toward your goals. Here's how to keep the fires of motivation burning:

-

**Visualize Success:** Regularly visualize your desired outcomes to maintain a clear picture of your goals.

-

**Review Your "Why":** Revisit the reasons why you set your goals in the first place. Remind yourself of your deep motivations.

-

**Adapt and Reframe**: Adjust your goals or strategies as needed, and see setbacks as opportunities to learn and grow.

-

Stay Accountable: Continue to engage with your accountability partner or mentor for ongoing support and motivation.

Your Progress and Motivation Action Plan:
Now, it's time to formalize your approach to celebrating progress and maintaining motivation. Follow these steps:

-

Goal: Write down the SMART goal you've been working on.

-

Celebration Milestones: Define specific milestones within your goal that are worth celebrating. Be as precise as possible.

-

Celebration Plan: Outline how you will celebrate each milestone. What rewards or activities align with your achievements?

-

Motivation Strategy: Detail how you will maintain motivation throughout your journey. How will you visualize success and remind yourself of your "why"?

-

Accountability and Support: Describe how you will continue to engage with your accountability partner or mentor to stay motivated.

By completing this action plan, you're setting the stage for a journey filled with positive reinforcement, enthusiasm, and the determination to persevere. Celebrating progress and maintaining motivation are vital elements in the pursuit of long-term success. In the upcoming chapters, we'll explore the role of adaptability and change as you continue on your path toward your goals.

Chapter 9: Embracing Change - The Role of Adaptability and Learning from Mistakes

Change is an inevitable companion on the path to success. In this chapter, we'll explore the importance of adaptability and the valuable lessons that can be gleaned from mistakes, helping you navigate the twists and turns of your journey with resilience.

The Necessity of Adaptability

Adaptability is the ability to adjust to new circumstances and challenges. Here's why it's crucial:

-

The Evolution of Goals: Goals may change as you learn and grow. Being adaptable allows you to modify your goals to align with your evolving aspirations.

-

Overcoming Obstacles: Adaptability equips you to overcome unexpected hurdles and setbacks.

-

**Maximizing Opportunities**: New opportunities may arise along the way. Being adaptable enables you to seize these chances for growth.

****Learning from Mistakes****
Mistakes are not roadblocks but stepping stones to growth. Here's how to extract valuable lessons from your missteps:

- _**Analyze and Reflect:**_ After a mistake, take time to analyze what went wrong and why. Reflect on the circumstances and your actions.

- _**Ownership:**_ Accept responsibility for your mistakes. Avoid the blame game and focus on solutions.

- _**Adapt and Adjust:**_ Use the lessons from your mistakes to adapt your approach. Modify your strategies to avoid repeating the same errors.

- _**Positive Mindset:**_ Cultivate a growth mindset, seeing mistakes as opportunities for learning and improvement.

Your Adaptability and Learning Action Plan:

Now, let's formalize your approach to adaptability and learning from mistakes. Follow these steps:

- _Goal:_ Write down the SMART goal you've been working on.

- _Adaptability Strategy:_ Describe how you will remain adaptable throughout your journey. How will you adjust your goals and strategies if circumstances change?

- _Mistake Analysis:_ Share an example of a mistake or setback you've encountered on your journey. Analyze what went wrong and what you learned from it.

- _Ownership_: Explain how you took ownership of the mistake and any steps you took to correct it.

- _Adapt and Adjust_: Outline how you adapted your approach or strategies based on the lessons learned from this mistake.

By completing this action plan, you're equipping yourself with the tools to face change and adversity with resilience and a growth mindset. Embracing change and learning from mistakes are integral components of your journey toward long-term success. In the following chapters, we'll explore the concept of perseverance and the role it plays in achieving your goals.

Chapter 10: Living a Life of Action - The Ripple Effect of Taking Action and Inspiring Others to Do the Same

Your journey of taking action is not just a solitary endeavor; it has the potential to create a ripple effect that touches the lives of others and inspires positive change. In this final chapter, we'll explore how your actions can influence the world around you and motivate others to embark on their own journeys of growth and achievement.

The Ripple Effect of Taking Action

Every action you take has the potential to create waves of impact far beyond your immediate circle. Here's how your actions can create a ripple effect:

-

Inspiration: Your actions can inspire others who witness your dedication and progress. They may see in you a source of motivation to pursue their own goals.

___*Leading by Example:*___ By taking action and persevering through challenges, you set an example of determination and resilience for those around you.

___*Community and Collaboration:*___ Your actions can foster a sense of community and collaboration, as others join you in pursuing shared goals and aspirations.

Inspiring Others to Take Action

Inspiring others to take action is a powerful way to contribute positively to their lives and the world at large. Here's how to inspire and support others on their journey:

___*Share Your Story:*___ Talk openly about your own journey, including the challenges you've faced and how you've overcome them.

___*Offer Guidance*___: Provide guidance, advice, and encouragement to those who seek it. Be a source of support and motivation.

___*Celebrate Others' Success:*___ Recognize and celebrate the achievements of others. Acknowledging their progress can boost their confidence and motivation.

___*Create Opportunities:*___ Whenever possible, create opportunities for collaboration and growth within your community or network.

The Ongoing Cycle of Action

Remember that the cycle of taking action is a continuous one. As you achieve your goals and inspire others, they, in turn, may become catalysts for change and inspiration themselves. This ripple effect can create a positive feedback loop, perpetuating the cycle of growth and achievement.

Your Action and Inspiration Plan:

Now, let's outline your plan for living a life of action and inspiring others to do the same. Follow these steps:

Goal: Write down the SMART goal you've been working on.

Ripple Effect: Describe how achieving this goal has the potential to create a ripple effect, inspiring others in your community or network.

Inspiration Strategy: Outline how you plan to inspire and support others in pursuing their goals and taking action.

Share Your Story: Briefly share your journey and the lessons you've learned. Consider how you can incorporate this into your strategy.

Celebration of Others: Describe how you will celebrate the achievements of others and create opportunities for collaboration.

By completing this action plan, you're not only enhancing your own life but also contributing to the positive growth of those around you. Remember that living a life of action is not a destination but an ongoing journey, and your actions can have a profound impact on the world. Continue to strive for your goals, inspire others, and watch as the ripple effect of positive change continues to spread.

Conclusion

Conclusion: Your Journey Towards a Life of Action

Congratulations on completing this journey towards a life of action! You've embarked on a path of self-discovery, growth, and transformation. As you reflect on your progress and newfound knowledge, let's recap the key takeaways from your journey:

- *The Power of Goals:* Setting clear, SMART goals is the first step towards turning your aspirations into reality. Goals provide direction and motivation for your actions.

- *Action Overcomes Procrastination:* Recognizing procrastination traits and taking the first step are crucial in breaking the cycle of inaction. Remember, action breeds momentum.

- *Consistency and Habits:* Building consistent habits sustains long-term success. Small, deliberate actions compound over time and lead to significant results.

- *Accountability and Support:* Accountability partners and mentors provide valuable guidance and motivation. Surrounding yourself with a supportive network can be a game-changer.

- *Celebrating Progress:* Recognizing achievements and maintaining motivation is vital. Celebrate your milestones and use setbacks as opportunities for growth.

- *Embracing Change:* Adaptability and learning from mistakes are essential skills. They allow you to navigate unexpected challenges and evolve with your goals.

- *Inspiring Others:* Your actions can inspire positive change in others, creating a ripple effect of growth and motivation throughout your community and beyond.

Remember, a life of action is a journey without a final destination. It's about continually seeking growth, pursuing your dreams, and making a positive impact. As you move forward, keep these principles in mind, adapt them to your evolving aspirations, and stay open to new opportunities and challenges.

Your journey towards a life of action is an ongoing adventure. It's about embracing each day as an opportunity to learn, grow, and make a difference. By taking action and inspiring others to do the same, you're contributing to a brighter, more fulfilling world for yourself and those around you.

Now, take a moment to celebrate your achievements and the knowledge you've gained. As you continue your journey, may you find purpose, fulfillment, and boundless opportunities for growth and success.

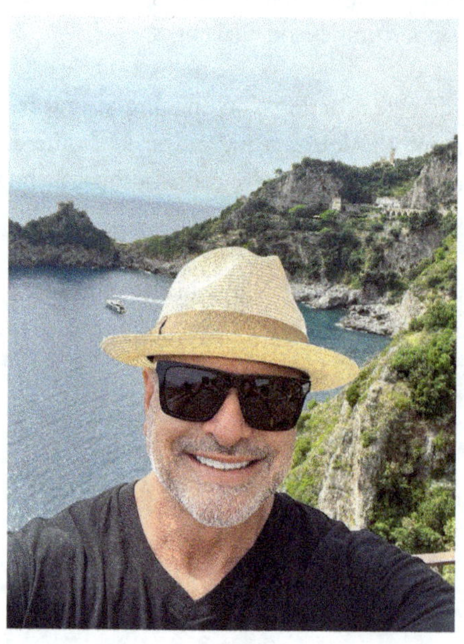

Dear Reader,

I wanted to take a moment to express my heartfelt gratitude for taking the time to read my eBook, The Art of Taking Action, Empower Your Life. Your support means the world to me, and I am truly thankful for your interest in my work. Writing and publishing an eBook is a labor of love and knowing that you chose to invest your time in reading it is incredibly rewarding.

Whether it was for entertainment, knowledge, or inspiration, I sincerely hope that you found value within its pages. It is empowering others to reach their goals, that I find the most fulfillment. If you are looking for support in your journey to health and wellness, please don't hesitate to reach out.

1Wishing you all the best, and I hope you continue to find joy and inspiration in the world of books and literature.
Warm regards,

John Bezerra